~ TABLE OF CONTENTS ~

Chapter One

~ The Way to Health ~

Growing up in a country town as a young boy, I would have to be in church at least three to four times a week. I can remember Tuesday night prayer service very well, because my father was the drummer and drove the bus for the church, and we would be at every service. On Tuesday, there would be a chair in the middle of the room, and everyone would be singing a church hymn that goes like: Come on in the room; Jesus is my doctor; he writes down all of my prescriptions; he gives me all of my medicine in the room. This song takes you out of the care of the medical men hands that were drugging and cutting, and places you in a natural condition to allow the body to heal itself; or surgery done without man's hands, but rather internal hands continually renovating and repairing the condition of the body. The chair symbolizes the act of pushing ones chair away from the dining table and placing it at the alter of mercy. Since the person is not using the chair for eating, it is used for prayer. The person can kneel down on the knees in prayer in the chair. Many people have received healing while following this service or ritual ceremony. The question is how does healing occur without the use of any outside source of medicine, herb, or treatment.

If we are to find health, we must first be a seeker of Her and walk into her room of healing. Prayer and meditation heals the mind, and fasting heals the body. In the Hebrew bible, we read that if one would seek they shall find. So, if we are not healthy in the body and mind, we are not seeking her. Instead, we are running after the things that destroy the body, and we think on things that corrupt the mind. These things are the cause of our dis-eases and dis-comforts. When we are stuck in a situation or trial, it's usually because we haven't learned from it, but have rather accepted it as our fate.

Growth is to become more mature in body, mind and soul. Again it is written in the Hebrew bible that the writer said that when he was a child he did childish things; but when he became an adult, he put away the childish things. To become an adult, you must put away childish things. To be healthy, you must put away all things that are unhealthy. Those things that destroy the physical body must be stopped, and the things that make the brain go insane must be changed to positive things to rather nourish it instead.

The natural state of humans is health. Only when we leave off of the path that leads to health do we suffer with dis-eases and dis-comforts. The path that leads to health must: be a clean and cluttered free place; have clean air to breathe; have pure water to drink; must have the type of food that promotes the greatest health; have a comfortable temperature; free of stress and violence; have adequate sunlight; plenty of time and places for rest and relaxation; ability to have mobility. The path that leads to dis-ease and sickness must: be filthy and attractive of parasites; have toxic air making it hard to breathe; have contaminated water to drink; have the types of foods that causes dis-eases and dis-comforts; have temperatures that are too cold or too hot; contain stress and violence; be in total darkness devoid of light; allow continuous movement with little to no rest or relaxation; allow continuous rest with little to no movement whatsoever. The unnatural state of humans is dis-ease. One path leads to health and the other to disease.

Uncleanliness is the state of not being clean, be it inwardly or outwardly. Imagine walking down a path that had a bunch of trash and filth all in the way. First, you would have the problem of movement do to filth. Second, the filth will attract insects and parasites. When your house is filthy and unclean, its first becomes hard to navigate around the house. Second, it becomes infested with parasites and insects. The insects came "'cause" of the filth and trash. The parasites and germs, as they eat and reproduce, they leave behind waste that is toxic to human cells. The waste must be removed from the body or placed out of the way of the vital organs. Energy is required in removing unnecessary toxins out of the vital domain. This takes away from other operations that require energy in the body. ALL CELLS REQUIRE ENERGY TO FUNCTION. This functioning power is called Nerve Energy. This waste adds on to the regular normal waste of metabolism. Uncleanliness causes the body to waste its precious energy supply in removing accumulating waste.

Cleanliness is the act of being clean, be it outwardly and inwardly at the same time the spiritual word 'holy' means whole, or sound body and mind. To have a sound body is to be clean inside and out. Washing the outside is great for outward cleanliness, but to have clean blood that builds the skin that you wash with water is of more importance. You keep waste out of the body by stopping the ingestion of poisons, and then by allowing the body to more efficiently rid itself of the toxins that it makes itself from the process called metabolism. The area around you should be clean, because the clean area will not produce parasites. There are no parasites because there is no rotting or decomposing going on. The parasites will leave toxic waste in your area to ingest and inhale in the air. Waste made or taken in into the body must be removed using up precious nerve energy. But when this nerve energy has reach a point of depletion due to the constant call upon its reserve, the organs that helps in eliminating the toxins will not have enough energy to function, which means that less toxins are being removed from the vital domain. The inside can be said to be unclean. If the accumulation continues, the body will search for and use alternative routes to eliminate the toxins. If there is no energy available for the elimination organs, the body will store the toxins in out of the way areas. Sometimes it uses organs that have been badly abused as a way to allow toxins to escape the body. The poisons irritate and kill healthy cells and attract parasitic organisms that cause more damage. In a clean environment a cell will flourish, as seen in the culture of the scientist; but in an unclean environment, cells are destroyed from their own waste production that was never removed, which attracted parasites, which came to eat you out of house and home. Only cleanliness can get you to health.

All humans are required to take in fresh air of oxygen. This air must be free of perfumes, soaps, lotions, deodorants, oils, air fresheners, candles, and etc. to breathe in the freshest air possible. Our windows should be allowed open at all times to promote a continuous stream of circulating air. Our work areas should be well ventilated. A lot of people have a tendency to go to gyms and never exercise in the fresh air. Most houses are energy efficient these days (This means that it is a sealed up box that neither air nor the weather can penetrate.) Imagine being in such a house with candles burning, air fresheners spraying every hour on the hour, the smell of pine and bleach on every surface, raw sewage coming from the bathrooms within the rooms, cooking, hairsprays, colognes, and other types of air toxins. All these things are being circulated in the limited air you have in your sealed box. The more you breathe in you extract what little oxygen is circulating; the more you breathe out will add carbonic gases to the circulating air. This means that the quality or cleanliness of the air is disappearing or changing with each breath you take in and out. In other words you are slowly suffocating yourself.

Some people didn't know that the body receives water in three ways: drinking water; receiving it through high-water foods such as fruits and vegetables; and when digestion takes place, hydrogen is a byproduct of proper digestion and we breathe in oxygen, and these two join together forming water(H_2O). The last two is witnessed greatly in the natural raw vegan. But let's understand our drinking water and how it can lead us on the wrong path to dis-ease. Pure water is tasteless, colorless, and odorless. It is void of everything except two parts hydrogen and one part oxygen (H_2O). It is used as a fluid in the body to make up all of its liquid needs. When this fluid is pure, it is used immediately in hydrating the cells of the body and keeping them healthy. The pure water aid in cleansing the body of waste by diluting it and transporting it out of the body. If the water is toxic with something other than hydrogen and oxygen, it can only transport the trash it brought in with it. Pure water is needed in keeping the body clean. A clean body is a healthy body on a healthy path to a long life.

Imagine being a builder building homes out of brick. All of the homes you build and repair is made out of brick. Let's suppose that all of the brick companies went out of business in your area, and you had to repair your old houses and build the new ones out of another material, namely straw. The patch work of the straw and the new houses build with the straw will not stand like the ones that were made out of brick. The body is a living organism requiring living material in which to repair itself. If living material is not available at the time of repair or building, the body will substitute with lower grade material. Any stress come upon the organism will cause it to fall due to its weak structure. The ideal food material that is living and suitable for the human construction is fresh wholesome uncooked fruits, vegetables, nuts and seeds. This should be eaten in moderation, when hungry, and when in a good mental state. If the food causes the body to build itself out of wrong materials causing its structure to become weak liable to dis-ease, then you are on the road to sickness and suffering. If you are eating raw fresh fruits and vegetables in moderation in good spirits, you're on the path that leads to health and a long life.

How many times have you, those who have experienced cold climates, came in from the cold paralyzed from head to toe? How many stomach and head freezes have you experienced from drinking ice cold drinks? Whenever the body's temperature drops too low, the body uses its precious energy supply to warm back to a temperature that promotes homeostasis (life.) Not only does the energy supply get depleted, but the production of heat produces waste and causes an internal toxicosis that needs to be removed using up more energy. Using up nerve energy unnecessary robs energy from other vital functions of the body causing them to fail in their actions. The same is true with hot temperatures. When we take hot showers or abuse the natural sun, the body sweats to maintain coolness. This cool down requires precious nerve energy to be used so that the body doesn't overheat and destroy its enzymes. Low nerve energy robs the organs of elimination of functioning power causing toxins to accumulate. This means that toxins will irritate the cells and cause parasites to set up home and feast off of the body. Normal temperatures do not lower energy and neither does it favor the production of parasites, thus leading us on the path towards health.

Imagine if you will a plant that is saturated with rain, or suffers from a drought. Imagine that plant taken out of good soil and placed in sand. Imagine the temperature so hot that the plant incinerates, or too cold that it freezes and die. Now, what happens to humans when these stresses are placed on them? Could it be that the energy of the body is called on to supplement the body's ability to handle the stress? This is a waste of the nerve energy, and if other energy depleting habits are present in the body, the body will rapidly reach a state of exhaustion or low energy causing toxins to accumulate in the body. The environment must be suitable for growth and repair. The relationships must be nurturing and not toxic. Being around someone who always makes you angry and upset will keep the internal environment toxic. Stress causes the fight or flight response to kick in. This adrenaline that is released in the cells to stimulate the cells to increased action. Increased action means increased waste production. Toxins accumulate in the body leading us down the path of dis-ease. There a hormone that deals with stress that the body produces call cholesterol. Chronic stress over produce this hormone causing elevated levels in the body. Nonstop production causes the body to produce a low-grade form of cholesterol to keep up with a steady production. This low-grade material will lump up and calcify in the body, causing blockage to the circulatory system. Anything that disrupts the natural operations of the body will cause its dis-ease or suffering. This is a path that is not recommended if one is seeking health.

The body must be strong and high in functioning power to deal with stress. The relationships that surround you must support your development and growth.

The sun should be taken in two forms: on the entire skin, directly through the eyes. Sunlight has a lot of benefits to our health and happiness. Picture the bat, he is blind because he never receive sunlight. You will suffer the same blindness if you live in darkness and never get sun. Dr. Kime wrote a book on the many benefits of the sun. He speaks about vitamin D produced when the sun rays mix with the natural oil and skin. Vitamin D helps with maintaining strong bones. Any element, mean, or influence will cause the body to become weak and unable to function correctly. Anything that weakens the body's energy will promote dis-ease.

Rest and sleep is the only way to generate energy. Energy is produced at a constant stream in the body. When the body is at full rest, more energy is being saved and not used in activity. When it is at full speed ahead or high activity, the energy is being depleted at a rate faster than the body can generate or produce. If you can recall, the organs fail in their work from lack of energy or fatigue. Imagine having a cell phone that runs on a twelve hour battery. The battery stays charge for 12 hours, and 12 hours is needed to recharge it for another full twelve hours of use. This is to only talk on the phone. However, if you decide to text or take pictures and talk, it will use up the battery in half the time, or 6 hours. If you decide to surf the internet too, the battery will only last 3 hours. The use time gets shorter as you do more things with the phone, but the charge time remain the same. Just like if you put the phone on the charger half full, it will only take 6 hours to charge. The human organism must connect to the universal charger called sleep to recharge its supply of energy. The less active the organism: the less need for rest. The more active the organism, the more it will need to rest. The more you use the phone, the more you need to have it charge. It holds a charge when not in use longer than when in use. In a healthy body there must be high energy levels. Rest and sleep allow the body to restore its energy levels at the fastest rate possible. This means that rest and sleep is needed to lead you on a path to health, because they restore energy allowing the body to operate with full functioning power. When all organs are functioning at optimum levels, this is considered health. No toxins can accumulate in a body whose elimination organs are operating at high speed with full power. Rest and sleep is necessary for health.

Now, it's one thing to not get rest, but another way to dis-ease is constant rest or laziness with no regular movement or exercise. A lot of us are suffocating in our own cellular waste. We have this fluid called lymph that is on the outside of the cell and on the inside. This fluid circulates through the body only by movement. If there is no movement, no lymph fluid will be circulated through the blood. This fluid is used in keeping the cells squeaky clean. The thing about it though, when no circulation of lymph fluid is in progress, the cells are not being clean. The waste that the cells make from everyday wear and tear are not getting wash away with the circulation of lymph fluid. The waste will soon irritate the cells to the point of death if lymph fluid is not constantly removed from the cells. Movement forces or squeezes the fluid out of the cell along with the cells waste. This toxic lymph fluid is taken and released into the blood system, and then it is removed from the blood by the organs of elimination before it is voided out of the body. This regular movement helps circulate lymph fluid that has been removed from the cells with the cells waste, and it dumps it into the blood system ridding the body of its waste materials. This means that regular movement is necessary to maintain clean cells. Clean cells mean that they will operate with the greatest efficiency. When cells operate at their greatest efficiency, this is what we called health. Remember, cleanliness is on the road that leads to health.

The germ theory of the medical men of today have

educated our minds into believing that germs are the only cause of our dis-ease. Hygiene teaches that the one cause of all dis-ease is 'TOXEMIA' or poison blood. This poison is an internal one. It is due to low nerve energy, which is due to excesses and abuses to the body. External toxins brought into the body that can be controlled are not, but rather wastes the body's precious nerve energy in cleansing them from the body. So, instead of removing the cells toxins from the body, the organs of elimination is constantly engaged in cleansing the external toxins that are allowed in the body out of it. This means that the cells waste are accumulating in the blood. The blood uses other routes to release these toxins out of the body (cold, flu, eczema, etc.) to keep the cells clean. But we go and take medicines or herbs to stop these routes or symptoms. Your medicine has just stop the cure of a toxic blood. The blood continues to be toxic since we stop the other routes of detox (cold, flu, eczema, etc.)The lymph is unable to dump its waste in the blood because it is already too toxic. So, the cells drown in their own waste. The waste irritates the cells to death. Death to the cell means death to the organism. This is the road to death when you actually destroy your own cells. At sometimes the body will build itself hard and tough to be able to withstand the constant irritation. However, this hardening changes the structure and function of the cells. In other words, your stomach won't hurt from irritation because it has harden, but neither can it squeeze and digest food. To save itself it has destroyed itself by becoming hard. This is what some would call stomach cancer.

Imagine a dirty trashcan full of waste. If left that way for a little time, Maggots and other parasites will appear. Now, imagine a clean trashcan without any waste, or waste constantly removed and cleansed. No parasite will bother to waste their time appearing. A landfill could never be a parasitic free environment. When we look at the human organism and its internal environment. If it is kept clean, no parasites will be attracted to it. But if it is swimming in waste, Parasites will make it stay there until they eat it out of house and home.

To travel the path that leads to health and long life, we must keep high nerve energy to keep the blood and lymph fluids clean so that the cells will remain clean. If the cells remain clean, they operate efficiently. This is what we call health. In restoring more energy into the body, we must avoid those things that rob us of our energy, and religiously apply those things that builds and saves our precious nerve power. These means and influences that leads to health are: a clean cluttered free internal and external environment; clean air to breathe; pure water to drink; the types of food that promotes the greatest health; comfortable temperatures; freedom of stress and violence; adequate sunlight; plenty of time and places for rest and relaxation; regular mobility.

Chapter Two

~ The Fall From Health ~

When the creation of man appeared on the earth at a time of unknown origin, his behavior was in complete compliance with nature. The air that surrounded him was that of pure air and not filled with toxins that exist in it today. The water was distilled by nature to not contaminate the fluids of the body. The air that invaded the lungs was not offending to its processes, neither were there clothes hiding the largest organ of the body as to not bathe in the benefits of the sun. Man did not know a toxic relationship or practiced addictive habits. His instincts were natural in nature. The rising of the sun woke man to a glorious day, and the twilight of the stars and moon tucked him to sleep on a ritual basis. Even though man seems to gorge his belly with any substance that is in his reach to consume, his original diet is that of a frugivore.

When we look at the changes that occurred from the earlier time of existence, we see that man's behavior has changed physically, mentally and spiritually. He no longer possess the vigor, endurance, and freedom from disease. His mentality has been condition by those powers that corrupt. His spiritual fall from nature has provided him a false hope in superstition.

Being, as supposed, the greatest of God's creation, Man has become a breeding ground of invalids. There are only few that carry the stature of structural health in its delightfulness. His upright stance has been traded for the bow in the legs, curvature of the spine, and protruding at the abdomen. His head is no longer aligned with the rest of his body. Instead of a model of excellence, man has become a host of cartoon characters.

The invention of the television has played a major part of man's fall from grace. This practice is a relative new one but is nonetheless a destructive one. He sits idle for hours on end staring at a screen that undoubtedly has him hypnotized, seeing the continual glare in his eyes and trance demeanor. Watching it usually hinders the flow of lymph fluid, and this will begin the accumulation of toxins in the body.

The television has a direct connection, or plug in, into the pre- frontal cortex, which is the CEO of the brain. Information is going in the brain, but no action is being taken at that precise moment. The viewer will act later as he passes McDonald's and realize "I'm Love n it". He will have no choice but to stop knowing he can have it his way.

Man is easily programmed! These advertisement agencies capitalize on this fact. Who can believe that an Olympic track star eats at McDonald's before his race? I see many who just want to go to sleep afterwards. Any chemist or physiologist knows that wrong food combination will render the eater lethargic. Take for example on Thanksgiving when after we've gorged ourselves on turkey, ham, rice, potatoes, pudding, cake and etc., what is the inevitable outcome? Sleep induced coma! With this being the case, why can't this behavior be changed?

For so long, has man been tricked or conditioned to behave a certain way. So many unknowing individuals would repeat something they learned from a blind teacher, a for-profit preacher, murderous physicians or fly by night "quack men". The doctors/teachers would say diseases are caused by germs. The preacher will accuse either God or some evil demon for man's suffering. The quack would say anything to fulfill his own gain.

The germ theory was put out by Louis Pasteur. Those people that follow his theory, such as allopathic doctors, believe that a foreign entity can at any moment invade the body and cause someone to become ill. They believe by heating up milk to a certain degree, it would kill the germs and bacteria that flourished in it. Not yet have they come up with a way to remove the dead germs/bacteria out of the milk!

If germs be the cause of disease, what activates a germ to invade the body? How does it start small and invade a strong immune system and make it weak; and, while it is in rapid reproduction of itself (the germ or bacteria), and able to do more harm; then gives up its fight and vicious attack, like we see of the common cold that we so call "catch." If dis-ease is caused by a weak immune, why do we behave from the medical mentality by trying to cure the cure! The sneeze is the cure, for the nose is releasing poisons through it. The cough is the cure: the mouth, lungs and throat is releasing toxins. This thought of curing the cure is a bad mental state of mind that has changed man's behavior to how he connects with nature.

The preacher man cannot be left out of this mental slavery that has shaped the behavior of man's thoughts and actions. With the thought of good spirits and the thoughts of evil one's, has produced a world of superstitious people. Instead of obeying the laws of God or nature, he resorts to ceremonies and witchcraft from the priests. He believes that praying will remove all his sicknesses and suffering while he continues to disobey the laws of his being. The naturalist speaks of some herb or plant that can take away man's suffering. If this being the case, we would be spitting in the face of God saying "we need not your law, for there is a way out." Why even make a law and provide a way out of each one? That doesn't make much sense to them that have been broken from this hypnotic trance produce by teachers of spirits as they teach from their pulpits!

These teachers that teach our kids at an early age are unlearned in the ways of life just like the rest. Our kids or snuffed up (by law, or jail will be the outcome) at an early age to sit idle in a classroom being taught the exact same information that has no bearing on life. Why do they not teach physiological nutrition? Why do they not teach the kids how to control their internal dialogue? How to control automatic negative thoughts? They teach discipline, but not self-discipline! Our children are exposed to hate in history, as it adds definition to their lives. No one can be afraid of the boogieman if they were never exposed to that story. In the Hebrew bible we come across a moment where God asks Adam and Eve who told them that they were naked.

As I stated earlier, we are creatures of habit. Whatever is programmed into our brain (the body's hardware) is the only information that is going to be able to be accessed. Just like a computer, whatever the programmer programmed on it, that's all you are going to be able to get it to do. If you wish to get it to do something else, you must get the software and upgrade new information on it. The computer at all times can be programmed and reprogrammed again. The type of software you put in it is the type of results you're going to get out of it. Nothing more and nothing less! The only change will result if the software crashes or the hardware breaks down.

If the brain is the hardware, what happens when it's not operating correctly? What happens when the machine is not working properly? What happens when it's not turning on? What happens when it's not getting a sufficient current or electricity, or a surge of electricity or activity? It doesn't matter how much software you place on it if the machine doesn't work. The best antivirus will find itself to be a complete waste of money and time if the motherboard is shot!

The brain being the storehouse of all information brought in and sent out, how does it alter the behavior of man if it is not working properly? Just like the computer; if regular maintenance is not performed; if physical damage is introduced on it; if excessive amounts of abuse is placed on it will make a crash a must. Would he not be able to process information? Would that information that he has be able to be exposed accurately? To be whole one must have a sound body and mind. The hardware must be acting right for the thoughts to be acting right. That will bring us right back to nutrition. The brain being a structural organ must abide by the laws of its organic nature. If that being the case: to be sound it must have the nutrition that is consistent with its nature. It cannot be replaced with parts that don't fit, or of a different caliber. It must have the elements that those cells are made of so it can repair and restructure itself with. It would be folly to patch a brick house with sticks, or a cement house with straw. If we do we must look out for the big bad wolf.

If we believe that health is only in eating, wouldn't our nation be the healthiest? Eating, we have no problem with. Matter of fact, we are a land of an abundance of food; we have so much that we are a wasteful nation. We are taught to eat in any situation. It doesn't matter if we're sick or well, we are encouraged to gorge ourselves with disease producing combinations, stay out of the night's air, stay away of the rays of sun, continue our self-destructive habits, encourage the ingestion of medicine, and follow superstitious practices. No one tells the individual to keep clean or get regular exercise. No one tells him to get sun or breathe pure air. No one tells him to eat the right foods or drink pure soft water. Neither does anyone tell him to get adequate sunlight and maintain normal temperatures. He even thinks that he can operate continuously without getting adequate sleep. His habits, unbeknown to him, are suicide habits. These are habits he can control, but not having the mentality to obey the laws of nature, his behavior points towards his destruction.

From the very onset of man's life, he has been endowed with an innate wisdom. However, through the course of time, he has lost his connection with nature. His behavior has been directed by pivotal people in the wrong direction for all the wrong reasons. This has caused plenty of disruption in the order of the universe. As long as he allows others to direct his path instead of the Author of nature, he will continuously be lead like a sheep to the slaughter.

Chapter Three

~ Natural Hygiene ~

Natural Hygiene is not the hygiene you receive from using a bar of soap; from brushing your teeth with toothbrushes and toothpaste; from the shampoos or deodorants. Perfect hygiene cannot be accomplished by lotions or oils. In fact, all those things that I have just named are artificial hygiene. They all are artificial means and methods to make the body appear to be healthy. You might say that there's an illusion that the person is in good health. Imagine a paint shop painting your car without sanding the rust and repairing the dents. Imagine the car owner who paints the car sanding and removing its dents with a blown engine that he refuses to fix, or doesn't takes the time out to fix. There are many who make-up and cover-up their blemishes and wrinkles, but never think to just repair the skin. The skin can radiate with beautiful radiance if it is cared for hygienically.

Natural Hygiene is when you allow the natural means and influences to promote health in the body. Medicines are not natural and neither are they means by which the body will heal. Medicines palliate symptoms of illness, but does nothing in correcting the illness or its cause or causes. If medicine had power of healing, it would have the power of action, for it will have to cause the body to act a certain way, and that certain way must be the same action every time regardless of who takes it . But we don't see medicines acting like that, or even acting at all. The body acts on the medicine according to its toxicity and the power that the body has on hand for itself to act in neutralizing and eliminating the medicine. The medicine is more of a direct threat to the vital organism than the dis-ease. So, the body's energy is redirected to neutralizing and eliminating the medicine that it stops repairing itself in the case of acute dis-eases, but in chronic diseases painkillers are the primary drugs in treatment. They can only put out the fire siren without being able to put out the fire. Natural Hygiene remove cause. Not only do it remove the cause of the fire, it makes the house fireproof.

If a medicine had any effect on health, it would have the same effect every time to anyone who took it. There would only be a need for one pain pill, if the pill had the power of action to control and stop pain. There will only need to be one laxative, if laxatives had the power of action to make the bowels move. It would also cause the same move with the same dose every time. But we see that to be not the case; the more you take the pain pill or laxative, the more is required next time to get the same action. This is carried on until the whole bottle can be taken without accomplishing any action. Then, the person is said to not be responding well to the medicine, but is better said that the individual has adapted or lost the ability to respond to the continual intake of the medical poisons. Just like when smoking a cigarette for the first time. Your lungs may respond violently with a rage of coughs until it acquires the fresh air it needs. This will happen again if you keep up the habit of smoking, but eventually the coughing will get less and less violent until you are able to smoke a pack a day without coughing one time. The body was acting on the smoke just like it was acting on the medicine. When the practice is continued, the body will adapt to any substance or habit before it allows its energy supply to reach a critically low point. It will accommodate any practice that is repeated. This means that at first entrance of poisons in the body, the body will fight vigorously to defend its domain; but after continuous warfare against the invading poison, and before its energy is depleted to the point of potential death, will stop fighting and allow the poison to have an all access pass into the vital domain without any opposition. This is the law of accommodation that Hygiene teaches.

So, it is the body that acts on these lifeless substances that we take in the hopes of curing our dis-eases and dis-comforts. This means that herbal, supplemental and other so-called 'natural' remedies are just as useless and destructive as the medicine man pills and potions. They all are the same but packaged and distributed by different medical mentalities. Notice that every school of health professional or healer today has a favorite remedy or treatment by which to sell you in exchange for your pocket book, and will have it available for your use to guide you with 'living' with your disease. None of them search out the cause of the suffering. They believe that swollen adenoids in the nose causes nose bleeds and snoring, and its cure is to remove the adenoids with surgery. I can see where snoring can be a symptom of a block nasal due to swollen adenoids, but why are the adenoids swollen? What are the adenoids? Are they not a part of the immune system? They are tonsils located near the rear of the nasal cavity that helps filter the air we breathe, trap and destroy microorganism. They enlarge to accumulate more microorganisms when more is present, and they enlarge when the drainage of the body is not functioning at optimum levels. Now we found the cause of a swollen adenoid, but what causes the slow drainage and accumulation of microorganism? Well, the body produces energy for you to deal with the environment and its stresses. We use this energy up in excess with our bad lifestyle habits, which that quickly depletes the nerve supply. So, when these wrong lifestyle habits are added to faulty elimination (when energy is low, the organs of elimination doesn't have the energy to detox and keep the body clean. This means that we are constantly on the verge of fatigue and full of toxins. Now, when a drop or rise in temperature, unusual exposure or an environmental stress places an added burden on the body, the body will not have enough of energy to defeat them both. The adenoids, along with the entire immune system, steps in and house the poisons from the body's vital organs and cells. If the load is great, the adenoid's tissues will expand itself to accommodate the toxins. However, this growth may be hazardous to the organs and tissue nearby. As the growth continues, space becomes more limited. This means that other organs will be pushed out of the way causing them to malfunction. So, cause or causes go way back to our lifestyle habits and environmental stresses. As we cannot control our environment in its entirety, we can control our lifestyle habits. This doesn't come to the mind of those who are in the business of curing and drugging.

Inflammation is not a cause of disease, but rather a response to any kind of insult or injury. It's usually a rapid general response to physical wounds, foreign objects, infecting organism, chemical toxins, heat or radiation. It is unlike the immune system, for the immune system responds with specific action from specific parts of the system to specific invading substances. The inflammatory response is a response that the body activates to send an increase of blood to an injured part to provide materials for repair of its damages and serves to protect the body from decomposing drugs and infectious matter. The more blood in that area, the more materials on hand for repair. But, this overflow of blood brings heat. The heat allows the metabolic enzymes to work faster in their repair work. The work of repair generates heat as well as the presence of more blood. The overflow of blood causes the area to swell. Why do we search to cure inflammation and not remove its cause? Imagine getting a tattoo, and the tattoo artist digs into your skin with his tattoo needle. You immediately feel pain and the spot starts turning red. Notice that the inflammation is a local one, meaning its location is only where the damage occurred. If you bruise the arm, the arm is inflamed and not the feet. If the feet is bruised, it inflames and not the arm. This means that where inflammation presents itself, there is some form of injury or invading poison created from within or taking in from without. Inflammation is not a disease in itself: but a means by which the body: repairs itself from injury and protect itself from harmful substances.

Hygiene teaches that the body is capable of healing itself, if healing is possible, when the cause or causes are removed. The environment must be favorable to its growth and development. The body has a monopoly on healing and will heal itself without any help from any medical or herbal man if its causes are removed and there is something still left there to heal.

The men of science teach us that there are laws of life that go on day after day that are fixed and unchanging. These laws helps us to understand the way nature work. Nature does nothing by chance. Instead, her work is based on a universal order that is eternal. Every living creature must obey these laws, for NO ONE is above the laws. The wild animals are born with an inner wisdom of instinct to obey the laws that govern their nature. No fish thinks he can live a life on land; neither do birds live a life flying in the deepest seas and oceans. Humans must obey laws too, but they lack instinct. They have to rely on their own intelligence to make sense of these laws to use them to their benefit.

One of the most basic of these laws is the Law of Preservation. Dr. Robert Walters (1841-1921) helps us to understand it by what he refers to as Life's Great Law: "Every particle of living matter in the organized body is endowed with an instinct of self-preservation, sustained by a force inherent in the organism, usually called vital force or life, the success of whose work is directly proportioned to the amount of the force and inversely to the degree of its activity." This means that every part in the living body, even to its smallest particle, has the will and ability to preserve itself without interruption due to an energy that is generated within the organism, which its success is according to the amount of the energy that is available.

So, every part of the body has a power called life in each individual particle, which will help it function according to the amount of this life that it has available at any given time. The cells of the human body will continue to perform their individual functions; which completes a whole to perform in harmony the best interest of the body as long as they are supplied with the power, means and influences necessary for its maintenance. These means and influences are: Cleanliness, fresh air, pure water, ideal diet, normal temperatures, adequate sunlight, rest and proper sleep, regular mobility and exercise, emotional balance and nurturing relationships.

When given these essentials, the on-board computer (brain) will do the rest. The life force is constantly working for the health and life of the body as long as life remains. The work it does is inherently built in and cannot be improved upon. So, the medicinal and herbal, treatment strategies are useless in trying to correct that which is already attempting to correct itself, according to the amount of energy it has to operate with. Hygiene proves that dis-ease is right action, meaning that the action is action that the body produces to rid itself of poisons and heal itself from injury. The body has a monopoly on healing itself. No other person can heal you but you. I cannot sleep, eat the right foods, exercise, get sun, keep emotional poise, and drink pure water for you. Each person must take this journey for themselves. Jesus of the Hebrew bible taught that each man must pick up his own cross and save himself. Imagine me healing you, you then belong to me because your health hang on my willingness to heal you. You then are my slave and I your master. I can produce health at will in you, or I can cause death in you. Hygiene teaches that the individual has the ability to heal itself where healing is possible. This meaning that you produce health and death in your own bodies by your own willingness and lifestyle habits. If you are diseased, you only need to examine your life and its habits to find its cause or causes. If you want health, all that is needed is that you stop the abuses and habits that are producing disease. Natural Hygiene is a science that teaches that health only comes from healthy living.

Chapter Four

~ Drainage, Nutrition and Vitality ~

Imagine having a pet fish in an empty fish tank, or imagine it being filled up with regular boiling hot faucet water. This fish is not in the environment needed for it to survive. It doesn't have a lot of the elements of its natural surroundings of ocean and sea life to a bowl of contaminated hot water. This will cause the fish to go belly up really fast. The fish would have lived out its normal lifespan if it was not taken out of its natural habitat and placed in a poison environment without any of the elements it need for survival. Humans suffer this same fate; however, we are the ones in charge of our own environment and needs. We place ourselves in environments that don't promote health and growth, but causes early unnecessary death. We drink liquids that are contaminated, hide from natural sunlight, eat foods that are not a part of our natural diet, refuse to get rest and sleep in complete quietness often, maintain excessive temperature, get plenty of toxic air, barely ever exercise, and always dealing with drama and toxic relationships. By doing these things, we are totally removed from what keeps us healthy, our paradise. This environment must be: clean, have fresh air and exposure to natural sunlight, clean distilled water, able to provide foods that promote health in the human, allow for regular mobility and exercise, quiet enough and allow rest, normal in its temperature, without stress, free from violence. If we place ourselves in such environments, we would live out our normal old lifespan with sound bodies and minds.

There is a law that states that, "Every cell of the body will continue to perform the function for which it was designed throughout its entire life cycle provided its environment remains congenial to it." If the nature that surrounds the cell remains in perfect condition for the cell to function, it will continue to function until the lifecycle of the cell ends. This is to say that there would be no early or premature death of the cell, and they would live out their entire life.

The human body is a community, or group, of cells that work together for a common cause, which is life. Instead of doing all the work required to maintain life in any one cell, their work is split, or divided up so that they specialize in what they do; and in doing so, they must rely and depend on one another to carry out its work efficiently. The cells form organs, which are special structures that perform special work: like the skin cells that protect from the outside world, the kidney cells that excrete waste, and parts of the liver that secrete bile or store glycogen. Even though some are special organs, there are fundamental functions that are common to all cells alike and are essential to the life of the cells. Doesn't matter how great or least a cell may be, there are functions that both, the great and the small and everything in between, will have to perform for the cell to have and maintain life. Systems are grouped to form the organism. Examples of a systems is: the digestive system: mouth, teeth, glands of the mouth and intestines and stomach, esophagus, stomach, liver, and the pancreas.

The amoeba cell is a single cell organism, and humans are complex organisms. By us being a complex of cells, the work of one part has a very important connection to the work of other parts. The lungs breathe oxygen for the heart, brain, and all the other organs and cells of organs. The digestive tract digest food for the entire body, for there is no other part of the human body that can perform the work of the digestive tract in digesting food material. The kidneys cannot do it, and neither could the reproductive organs digest any sort of food item. Once the germ cells of the developing embryo decide or choose which organ or structure it's going to take the form of, it can never go back to being any other thing other then what it took on to be in the beginning of the embryo. Once the cells decide to be heart cells, they cannot change to any other cell. They cannot decide not to be a heart anymore, but instead choose to be a lung, kidney or liver.

Under normal conditions the amoeba is said to possess

eternal life, or not be able to die. Unless it is poisoned or starved, the amoeba is witnessed in the laboratories to go on dividing and dividing forever. Even when men of science experiment in the laboratories with pieces of tissues from animals they have found that if these are washed clean each day and supplied with a fresh nutrient medium or solution, they are able to live indefinitely. In nature we see that trees and plants live as long as their environment is favorable for it to have life. If the plants and trees are poisoned from pollution or starved from unfertile soil, the trees and plants will have died because the means and influences needed for it to live is not available, or those things that stops it from living is present.

The cells of the body require, if they are to continue to have life, grow and reproduce, proper nutrition, adequate sunlight, a normal temperature, and protection from violence. Cells, in the men of science laboratories, are killed by starvation and poisoning. If this is the only means by which to kill cells in the laboratories, why don't we conclude that this must be the same way cells are killed in the body? The cells in the body is constantly exposed to toxins from daily cellular activity, and from toxins that are absorbed from without the body. We poison ourselves daily from just breathing and other processes that carry on in the body. We bring in poison from external sources from our lifestyle habits and the environment that we live in. Drugs, vaccines, antitoxins, and etc., kill cells and cripple organs. Starvation of the cells are from eating foods that doesn't supply the body with the vitamins, minerals, or other nutrients that it needs. Impaired digestion from wrong food combining, or other abuses to the digestive system: starve the cells from getting the food nutrients it needs. If the tract is not working correctly, no food is getting digested properly. Undigested food cannot be used for the body, but is actually toxic to the cells. They are toxic because they are useless and in the way.

Life processes are performed ideally only in a nutritive medium when in a state of a liquid solution. Imagine the blood being a solid, How would it circulate and transport materials to the many cells of the body? How would it pick up the waste and drop them off to the elimination organs to be voided? The amoeba lives in water, animals have blood and lymph, and plants and trees have sap. The medium, or liquid solution, bathe every cell in the body and acts as a common carrier for all the cells. It supplies them with food, oxygen, and removing their waste.

In humans, only the lymph comes in direct contact with the majority of the cells and is constantly being replenished by the blood. The lymph picks up the waste that the cells produce from wear and tear. It circulates to the blood and mingles with it along with the waste. The blood transports the toxins to the organs of elimination to be voided. The circulation of lymph is increased with movement. Regular mobility and exercise will speedily circulate lymph and cleanse the cells keeping them squeaky clean.

Life in a complex organism depends on proper nutrition, correct drainage, and a good supply of nerve energy or functioning power. Without proper nutrition, the body would starve. Without correct drainage, the body will be poisoned with its own waste. Without functioning power, there is no power to do anything.

Nutrition is the digestion, absorption, assimilation, and dissimilation of food, water and oxygen. People actually believe that food is nutrition alone. Like food is the only influence on the organism development and growth. They don't think that water, sun, rest, and other factors help in the health and growth of the body. What good is eating the healthiest foods, while breathing toxic fumes? What good is breathing fresh air while ingesting poisonous food?

Drainage is the body's way of removing waste and toxic matter away from the cells and tissues by the blood and lymph and sent to the elimination organs and then voided. Imagine living in a house. Suppose that you generate a garbage bag full of trash every day. What would become of the condition of the house if you take out a full garbage bag out every day? How about if you take out one full garbage bag every two days? What if you don't take out the trash at all? Not taking out the trash will cause the trash to accumulate at a rapid rate. This will cause a filthy living environment for you to live in. The garbage will decompose and rot causing death to the cell. The cells of the body must be kept tidy and clean if they are to function properly. These cells produce waste from their work. The waste must be removed from the environment of the cell. The more waste removed, the cleaner the environment is going to become. Life comes from clean cells and death comes from poison cells.

Innervation is the constant and regular supply of nervous energy or nervous impulse to the organs and tissues of the body. If the nerve supply to an organ or part is destroyed, it loses sensation and motion and perhaps it will shrink or become smaller but not necessarily die. However, organs cannot function without the presence of nerve energy. Imagine eating, again, the healthiest of the healthiest of foods with a stomach that doesn't have the energy to digest the food eaten. The food will remain in the stomach longer than allowed, causing the food to rot and decompose. Without energy, there is no action. The body runs on a hygienic concept called "Nerve Energy." This nerve energy is generated by the brain. The energy is generated fast when the organism is not active or sleep, and the energy is rapidly depleted faster than it can be generated when the organism is active and awake. This energy can be used, or saved and stored for emergencies. It can also be depleted to the point of a critical low level or to a point of exhaustion. If this energy reaches a low energy level, elimination organs are among the first organs to lose function. This means that the toxins that the body produce and take in from without will not be removed from the blood and cells. This is terrible drainage. If the organs that helps drain the poisons out of the body can't drain the body of its waste, the cells and tissue will drown in their own waste and filth. This is what hygiene calls an autointoxication.

Energy is needed for both, nutrition and drainage. Energy is needed in digesting, assimilating, chewing, and all other areas of nutrition. Energy is also needed for drainage. Proper nutrition helps maintain high energy without the poisoning of toxic food items. Nutrition is needed to feed and fuel the organs and processes that drain the toxins from the body and keep the cells clean and new. Proper draining allow the body to conserve its energy, by having healthy cells to generate the energy. The one require the others, and the others require the one. Proper nutrition, correct draining, and functioning power will keep all the many cells and parts working properly.

Chapter Five

~ Build a Shack or Mansion? ~

In the Hebrew scripture, we find that the only way God would live in the temple was if it was holy. He would depart when any uncleanliness persisted. The temple is better said the human body, for it is the only temple made without hands, but rather made through a biological process of metabolism. This process is the process of life. The body can be made strong, or it can be made weak or not at all. The body can be said to be similar to the spacesuit of the astronaut. For the astronaut to survive on another planet, they must occupy a special suit, between them and the environment that adapts them to that environment. Imagine the horror in learning that an astronaut, while on mars, ripped his spacesuit constantly and never took the time to repair it. The astronaut goes day after day allowing the spacesuit to rip until it burst at the seams and falls all off. Here, on Earth, we have what we call an earth suit (body) that protects you from the environment. We've witness the horror of humans abusing their bodies constantly and never taking the time out for rest and repair. No matter how bad we feel, we just go on eating, drinking, working, playing and all other energy depleting habits. We keep producing and manifesting different dis-eases and dis-comforts until they cause our death.

The earth suit is stitched out of living thread unlike the manmade spacesuits.

The body is similar to a house. If the maid of the house is sorry and lazy, the house will become cluttered and full of filth. This filthiness will cause parasites to appear, like roaches, maggots and termites. The parasites will eat the filth along with the structure of the home inside and out. The house is then said to be uninhabitable or condemned. It becomes an eyesore and soon enough knocked down and used for scrap pieces and thrown in the landfills and junkyards. If we fail in the duties of taking care of our health, our body becomes toxic and low on vitality or functioning power. This accumulated waste is food for parasites, which migrate or appear in the human organism. As they feast on the waste, they will destroy anything in their path. The human is then said to be sick or diseased. The body deteriorates and becomes run down. The body will be placed shortly in the cemeteries and graveyards. The house is your body; and the filth is toxins that have been accumulated from wrong living habits. The roaches, termites, and maggots are viruses, bacteria and others types of pathogens. YOU ARE THE MAID!

Before the science man came up with his viruses, germs, and bacteria, the religious men would place the blame of their sicknesses and discomforts on God's wrath, the Devil, or his demons. They never thought for a second that their dis-eases and dis-comforts were built by their own bad lifestyle habits. It is as if a drunk man believes another person, or thing, is the cause of their stumbling and not his own alcohol poisoning. When he drinks alcohol, the body uses its precious nerve energy to neutralize and eliminate the poisons out of it before the organism is poisoned to death. When this energy is continually abused along with some other bad habits, the energy supply of the body reaches a critically low level. Organs and tissues that were usually receiving full nerve or functioning power are now having to settle with a fraction of the energy it was used to.

The elimination organs are first to lose function or functioning power. The kidneys don't filter the blood efficiently, or the bowels become constipated not releasing its contents. The more these elimination organs function less, the more toxins build up in the body. As the toxins continually keep building up, the body is being poisoned to death. To save itself, it finds an alternate route of escape for the toxins. This route may be the weakest organ or tissue of the body. This route is usually an uneasy and uncomfortable one. Some call these routes dis-eases and dis-comforts.

God doesn't weaken nerve energy, and neither the devil or his demon friends. Our bad habits lower nerve energy. Lowered nerve energy causes the body to accumulate toxins that are unable to be eliminated due to the low functioning power of the elimination organs. These toxins are irritating to the living cells of the body, thus causing the body to forcefully remove them from its environment. This process may be painful, uneasy, and uncomfortable. According to the danger of the toxic load will determine the severity of the dis-ease. If the toxic load is not so high and threatening, you may experience a slight drip from the nose. If the toxic load is high and threatening, you may vomit, have a diarrhea, or eruption on the skin.

When our hair turns grey, we die it with color. When we develop wrinkles, we find creams and the surgeon's knife. Instead of stop eating, we have the butcher chop off a portion of the stomach to control our eating. We lotion ourselves, and use all kinds of artificial outward hygiene covering up all of our blemishes from our bad lifestyle habits. The blemishes don't need covering up; they need to be repaired and rejuvenated. Imagine having a house that has recently been infested with termites. Every day you go outside and place a fresh coat of paint on the trimming of the house and scrub the bricks and driveway. You keep the lawn cut trim and watered. You go on day after day in this manner allowing the termites to continue infesting the inside. Those who walk by will swear that the house must be beautiful inside, but little do they know that the house is being eaten from within. Nothing within is being done about the termite infestation. There will soon be no more wood left in the house to paint when the termites gets done. What good is make-ups, oils, lotions and perfumes etc.? The body is built from the inside and not from the outside. Growth is a biological process or life process, and is accomplished only by the body. Imagine having a car that you regularly wash, polish and buff daily. You put expensive paint jobs, rims and tires on it often to change its look. You have a marvelous sound system installed, and redo the tint on the windows monthly all with a major short in the electrical wires and engine with a blown head; or cracked radiator. What good is it in putting all your time and money into the outer appearance of a car that can't be driven without first having an overhaul?

The body builds itself according to the grade of material (food) that is available at the time of building (anabolism.) It also builds itself according to the amount of functioning power (energy) it has at the time of building (anabolism.) Imagine being a carpenter, and you need to build a house before the week is over. It takes ten men to build a house in a week. For you to build this house in a week, you need nine other men to help you. If you hire only eight men to help you, you will not finish the house in time and you won't get paid. If you hire eighteen men, the house will be done in half the time. For you to finish the house on time, you must also have all the materials that are needed to make the quality of structure that is of the highest grade. If you don't have shingles and bricks for the workers to finish the house, you will have wasted money on labor because there were no bricks to build. You need sufficient manpower and the best materials to build the best building in a reasonable time. Without the manpower, the material cannot build itself. Without the material, the builders have nothing to build; or will use materials that are of a lower grade building a structure of lower quality. Instead of a mansion, it will be a shack. You need sufficient functioning power and the best materials needed to keep the human body healthy and full of vitality. Without functioning power, the food cannot digest and turn itself into blood, bones and flesh. Without food, there is nothing to turn into new blood, bone and flesh.

If you are giving your body the best materials and have the energy available to use the material in repairing itself, healing and repair will take place. Materials don't build the house, but the workers shape the materials into a mansion or shack according to the grade of material and energy available to the building process (anabolism.) Food, sun, water, exercise and mobility, emotions, air and temperature are all means and influences that the body uses to repair and build itself. So, the body is the healer and the natural things that help in keeping the body healthy is the materials. Cleanliness, pure water, clean air, adequate sunlight, ideal diet, normal temperature, regular exercise, rest and relaxation, emotional balance and nurturing relationships are the means and influences that saves the precious energy from being used up to be used for repair and building (anabolism.)

Should we build a shack or a mansion? Should we continue to use make-ups and cover-ups to hide our blemishes and conditions of the internal environment? These questions remind me of an old story of a beautiful young lady who everyone loved. She was so loved that she didn't have to worry about locking her doors. One day a knock came to the door, and she yelled for them to come in since the door was never locked. When the door open death was standing there looking at her face to face. When she realized that it was death, she started pleading to him that she was not ready to die. Death assured her that this was merely a visit because he was picking up her neighbor who was sick for quite some time. She sighed a sigh of relief and asked him to send her a sign or warning when he was returning to her, and he agreed. Years went by and the lady face started to wrinkle. Her sight starting growing dim: and her hearing starting getting bad. Her teeth started to fall out along with her grey hair. She used creams for the wrinkles in addition to the surgeon's knife. She wore glasses and received a hearing aid from the medical men. She even visited her local dentist to get some false teeth to replace the real ones. She was trying to cover and make-up every sign and warning of death without correcting the cause of the dis-eases and dis-comforts.

As she set in her chair and stared in the mirror, a knock came to the door. As everyone thought her to be so beautiful, she was so loved that she still had no reason to lock her door. So, again, she yells for them to come inside. When the door opens, death is once again standing in the doorway. She is surprised to see him without any sign or warning of his return. So, she asks him who in the neighborhood he was coming to pick up. He told her that he was there for her this time. She was taken off guard with what he told her, but he went on to explain to her that he sent many signs and warnings of his return, but they all was ignored and covered up.

In the Hebrew bible, we read that man should remember the creator in the days of his youth and before the troublesome days come. The lady was going on with her life neglecting the creator (builder) and maintainer of her life to false health and repair of her malfunctions. She had a visit before from death, but wasn't on the list to go. Most of us has had diseases that felt like death, but that's just death warning us to examine our lives and see what is luring him to come to us. After repeated signs and warnings have been given, the colds and other acute dis-eases turn into more chronic dis-eases. The body starts to fall apart and death is there to take you away. We cause death to come to our house. We all know the fate of a flower that requires water and sunlight, and if it is void of these to it will start to slump over, dry up, and wither away. Is there something to substitute sunlight and water to keep the plant alive and bearing fruit? No. It is equally true that there is no substitute for the means and influences such as: cleanliness, pure water, clean air, adequate sunlight, normal temperature, ideal food, emotional calmness, rest, regular exercise and nurturing relationships. A bandage can cover up the wound, but it is still there and must wait on the body to heal and close it up. Wounds heal with and without bandages, so the body is present in both healings, but the bandage is not. This can only mean that the healing process is done by the body and heals with or without treatments, so treatments are unnecessary. The cause of the wound must be stop before healing can occur though.

Imagine scraping your hands on a rough paved ground, and you irritate your hand to the point that it is bleeding. As long as you continue scraping, the wound will continue to bleed until it builds calluses and hardens. This hardening tissue is not premium or high-grade tissue. The low-grade tissue does not function as well as the high-grade tissue. This means the vitality of the person has developed a handicap.

Covering up the outside while we are dying on the inside will soon enough get you a visit or a one way trip with old death. Clean up the inside by cleaning its blood. Clean your blood by things such as: eating less; Eating the kinds of foods that supply the best material for the body without using up all of its nerve energy in turning it to blood, flesh, and bones; allow yourself to get sufficient sunlight on the bare skin; wear clothes that are light in color and loose on the body; Use pure clean distilled water to drink when you are thirsty; breathe in deep and often; get as much fresh air as possible; Keep your body at a comfortable temperature(not too cold or not too hot); exercise one to three times a week; Keep your emotions in check; keep a will to live; remove yourself from people who causes you to get upset, mad or angry; get as much rest as the body demands of it.

When getting rest, it is better to be lying down in a dead position like when laying in a coffin. This should be the position while breathing in deep through your nose and out of your mouth. For better rest, inactive standing is better than light work; sitting is better than inactive standing; lying is better than sitting; laying down sleeping is best of all for rest. Rest and sleep is the only means of building and restoring energy. The more energy generated by the body, the more energy will be available for repair and maintenance.

Nutrition is not just food, but it is every mean and influence that ends in what we call 'LIFE.' Imagine yourself eating fresh wholesome organic apples, and imagine eating this food in a room without oxygen. Think about how it will be to get sleep while lying in a fire. Nutrition is the sum total of all the natural means and influences that the body uses in building and repairing itself. It uses the sun for Vitamin D to build stronger bones, and uses water to replenish the body fluids when used by the sweat glands, urine and other liquids that escape from the body. If complete nutrition is not available during building and repair work, the body can only use what it has available. Imagine owning a car manufacturing plants that build cars. You have enough tires to build ten cars, but other materials are enough to build a hundred cars. We can only build according to the sum total of all the materials needed in building cars. The rest of the material is useless without having tires to put with them. It doesn't matter the part, if it is vital in the operation of a car, then car building is limited to the amount of parts that are in the least amount of parts in inventory. This is called the law of the minimum in natural hygiene. Can you make ten quarts of Kool-Aid with one packet that makes only two quarts? What if you had one quart of water? Ten quarts of water and five packets that makes two quarts each are required to make ten quarts of Kool-Aid. Any shortage in one will cause a weak drink, or a drink too strong and less to drink. When complete nutrition is on hand, the body will build itself evenly for the greatest health.

When we build ourselves with the greatest materials, we are reassured that our earth suits are strong and that they will keep us safe on this planet we call earth. If you was on Mars, you would have to be able to survive on that planet by being dressed accordingly and having the necessary apparatuses (organs) that helps us to deal with Mars environment. By us being on earth, our suit is a living suit called a body. Its organs helps us to operate and live in earth's environment, and to purify us of any impurities that threatens or jeopardizes the integrity of the suit (body).

It is a big deal that you live in such a way that you will be strong enough to deal with the earth's environment. Making sure to maintain cleanliness; breathing in the purest air possible as deep as you can as often as you can; drink purified distilled water according to your need for it; get lots of natural sunlight; eat fresh uncooked fruits, vegetables, nuts and seeds; get some regular exercise weekly; try to maintain a room temperature in all areas of your life(food, drink, bath, environment, etc.); get rest and relaxation; keep yourself calm and poised in your emotions; only keep positive people around that make you happy. Instead of embracing our sicknesses, as is the custom right now, we should embrace a possibility of living forever.

Chapter Six

~ Herbal Cures and Remedies ~

At an early age, I decided not to allow the doctors to dose me with their man-made poisons. For along time, before, I allowed the medicine men to practice their art of medicine destroying my body. I was previously on three different types of prescriptions for diverse illnesses. These medications did nothing to correct my situation, except the illusion that health comes with each swallow. With doctors out of the way and a continued bad habit, I was still in a dis-eased state. This dis-eased state caused me to pursue in a search for an herbal "cure" or "remedy."

This pursuit led me on a journey to stop the sickness and illness that was destroying my body. I searched many schools of healing in search of this so-called cure. At this point in my conscience, herbs were my truth. I felt that there was some plant or tonic that would take away any suffering of my body. This statement soon would be proven a "false" one.

Even before I came into the knowledge of Natural Hygiene, I was seeking to become a Master Herbalist, even after all my personal experience with these herbs in my own health conquest showed no improvement; they actually proved toxic to my health. Furthermore, I watch countless regulars frequent a health food store purchasing their magical potions only to grow weaker physically and develop emotional weakness from believing one is doing his/her best only to fall deeper and deeper into sickness. The cost of these herbs and supplements could run high, causing financial destruction. It is foolish to think that health is something to be bought rather than obtained by obeying the laws that govern us. Most prices were more than it cost to actually buy, the fruits or vegetables that contained them.

The use of Herbs goes back a long way. The shaman priest and the witchdoctors would supply their test subjects with this natural found in nature substance that would ward off unclean spirits. It would cause vigor in the weak; calm the nerves of the jittery; stimulate a lax nervous system.

The most common way to obtain herbs in an attempt to use them for some so-called 'curing' nature is at a retail store. When we go to these natural health food stores and purchase their herbal remedies, we are relying our faith of healing to those scientist and, cooperation's in its production. These herbs have plenty of toxic affects that we mistaken for healing. We can take Senna for an example. Senna is a potent cathartic, in measured amounts, a common ingredient in many proprietary laxatives. Senna is practiced as a cathartic drug, and is based on its content of so-called dianthrone glycosides, principally sennosides A and B with lessor amounts of sennosides C and D, as well as other closely related compounds. These are toxic to the body, so the body finds the fastest and least harmful route to get rid of these toxins. The action of the body forces the bowels to act and empty the toxins that were sent to it from the body. So happens, everything that occupies the bowels is released in this action. The toxic irritation of this herb has caused the bowels to empty it from the body. This is a forced action that will undoubtedly adhere to the law of limitation. The laxatives of the medicine men, and them of the herbal men, is that one is more toxic than the other; but that too, can be debated. The more toxic an herb is; the more the herbalist proclaims its curative properties. Habitual dosing with this or any other anthraquinone - containing laxative, and excessive irritation of the colon will result. Chronic abuse may cause electrolyte disturbances and fluid imbalances due to potassium loss and may interfere with or potentiate the activity of cardiac glycosides. It is clearly obvious that it would better serve all to stay clear of these natural poisons.

The research money and time is a reason to object to the use of herbs. Medicine patents cannot be placed on nature. Only chemical concoctions and witch pot breweries can obtain patents to profit from their tonics of death. Pharmaceutical companies are not going to spend large sums of money to research an herb that can be sold by anyone. They would not have sole rights to its profits. They would be doing the groundwork for everybody that wished to make money from it. These herbs have not had the proper research time due to the fact of low research money. Low money means that fewer scientists and other means of research will be limited to its attention.

Now, looking into the little research that has been done, we find that these herbs are thought to be a treatment for a wide range of ailments. Why? Because the body's rule of self-preservation diverts its nerve energy from a simple toxin removal process to a more urgent emergency removal of these poisonous herbal stimulants. Thus, the dis-ease is ignored until the body has successfully neutralized the toxic effects of the herbs. Therefore, the more toxic the herbal stimulant, the more nerve energy is going to be diverted to neutralize it. The more nerve energy is diverted; the less energy is going to be used for the dis-ease (abnormal elimination using abnormal routes).

Let us look at Mullein. It is thought to be valuable in the treatment of a wide range of ailments. When these herbs are hailed to such a degree, it makes them the newest "wonder drug." Notice the word drug in its praise. It is believed to possess demulcent, emollient, and astringent properties and is useful in treating both, bleeding of the lungs and of the bowels. It sedates and possesses narcotic properties, and it is thought to be useful in treating asthma, coughs, and hemorrhoids. Burns, bruises, frostbite, diarrhea, ear infections, and migraines are thought to be cured by Mullein. This drug is taken internally, applied locally, and even smoked, to treat these various conditions. Once the illusion is taken from our minds, we find that these herbs work in the same manner as does the murderous medicines of the allopathic school of healing.

To set our attention on natural herbs as a curative agent

is an erroneous one. When we think that we are finding new plants and introducing them to the world as a "new" wonder drug, we need only do the research on its use in prior generations. We would quickly learn why these other generations soon lost their faith in these voodoo practices.

Papain, which is vegetable pepsin, which is a mixture of proteolytic enzymes with a broad spectrum of activity; it hydrolyzes not only proteins but small peptides, amides, and some esters as well. Other components of the crude enzyme mixture hydrolyze both carbohydrates and fats. This wide range of activity accounts for the use of Papain in herbal medicine. Face- creams, lotions, cleaners, and so on are often formulated with Papain in the belief that the enzyme will exert "a digestive effect on freckles and other sun blemishes" while cleansing the pores of makeup and providing a general "softening" effect. However, a more familiar use for Papain is known by housewives as a meat tenderizer. The enzyme mixed with salt, which is a protoplasmic poison, as an activator and a carbohydrate-dispersing agent is sold in every supermarket. When we shake this on tough meat before cooking, it acts as an effective tenderizer by predigesting to some degree the fibrous animal protein. If this herb breaks down animal protein where they are in each other's presence, then what would become of the protein of the human animal? Would it not proceed it digesting it also? This is one of the very reasons why the body must direct total attention in expelling these toxins so that it is not digested from these destructive poisons. Once the toxins are eliminated, the wisdom of the body will redirect its energy to maintenance.

Keller lists more than sixty different ailments for which sage is claimed to be therapeutic. These range from aches to wounds and include such conditions as congealed blood, falling sickness, insomnia, measles, rheumatism, seasickness, venereal disease, and worms. It is highly probable that every sickness known to man will be listed as being 'cured' by sage. Sage cannot be recommended as a medicinal for internal use because of its high thuyone content. Details of the poisonous character of thuyone can be learned researching on wormwood. Basically, it can cause both mental and physical deterioration when consumed in small amounts over a long period of time. Large doses can result in convulsions and loss of consciousness, which are not desirable curable properties.

Let us look at milk thistle to be an all cure. It has been used for many years for a variety of conditions. It's praised was short lived in the early twentieth century just to have a couple of modern day charlatans to raise it's evils from the dead.

These are considered herbal diuretics: Angelica, Borage, Broom, Buchu, burcock, calamus, celery seed, chicory, cucurbita, dandelion, horsetail, hydrangea, juniper, lovage, mormon tea, parsley, rosehips, sarsaparilla, saw palmetto, and uva ursi. It is amazing that the herbalist has a wide range of herbs here. These are considered digestive aids: calamus, capsicum, catnip, celery seed, chamomile, dandelion, gentian, ginger, goldenseal, horehound, juniper, myrrh, papaya, parsley, pennyroyal, peppermint, peppermint oil, pollen, rosemary, sage, and savory. With all these herbs, the herbalist cannot curve what correct food combining can eliminate.

Am I to believe that aloe, boneset, cat's claw, Echinacea, garlic, propolis, schisandra, and suma will enhance my immune system? Can I be restored to health while I continue with un-cleanliness, impure air, impure water, irregular exercise, improper foods, abnormal temperatures, emotional imbalance, toxic relationships, inadequate sunlight, and lack of rest and relaxation? No! The immune system is what is needed to eliminate the very same herbs the herbalist sells to you. Therefore, you are actually weakening your system even more. Why attempt to fight dis-ease without first removing its cause or causes. The herbal mentality is no different from the medical mentality. They both believe that the living can be cured by the medicinal action of poisonous substances. Some are just high priced placebo's that are making its pusher rich. The curative action that they are so ascribing to these substances is one that should only be ascribed to the living, which has the power of action. Herbs are actually nothing more than an energy depletion practice, because the body is going to have to deplete its energy in expelling the harmful herb.

Whenever herbs are used to diagnose, cure, mitigate, treat, or prevent disease, they are, by definition, drugs. They do not possess magical or mystical powers that the herb-man would make you believe; and, like other drugs, herbs must be administered in proper doses for appropriate periods to produce their benefits. Every herb is different from every other herb, and as is the case with other drugs, their administration may produce undesirable side effects.

The widespread belief that plant remedies are "naturally" superior to man-made drugs has produced a wave of enthusiasm and promotion on the part of the public that can only be described as an herbal renaissance. Most of the people who are following this movement are more enthusiastic than knowledgeable about natural healing. Most people still harbor some of the medical mentality still. They have not fully changed their awareness to upright health. They are still looking for a curing application. These herbs could be sold legally if they were not labeled for use in the treatment of disease. Most labeling, books, and pamphlets carry a carefully worded disclaimer in directing that the reader should refrain from testing any of the suggested remedies but, instead, should consult a physician on all matters pertaining to drugs and therapy. We are given a bunch of information and then told not to apply it. There is literature that recommends large numbers of everything herbs for the treatment anything. These herbalists are recommending dangerous, even deadly, poisonous herbs on the basis of some outdated information.

Burdock is primarily used as a blood purifier, but has

also been used to treat various chronic skin conditions, including psoriasis and acne. It is also said to have diuretic and diaphoretic properties. None of these purported effects has been verified by clinical trials, nor have chemical studies of the root revealed the presence of active principles that might account for any such effects. Now, commercial samples of burdock are prone to adulteration with the root of belladonna, or deadly nightshade. The roots of these plants closely resemble each other, and confusion often occurs. Being this the case, it seems reasonable to insist that marketers of burdock test their product and certify that it is free from belladonna contamination. However, no solid evidence exists that burdock exhibits any useful therapeutic activity.

Catnip contains a volatile oil that is extremely attractive to cats, causing them to cavort playfully while attempting to saturate their entire bodies with the plants distinctive aroma. Catnip was once rather widely used in human medicine, primarily as a carminative or digestive aid, and as a tonic. The hot tea taken at bedtime has been recommended as a sleep aid, and most of its enthusiasts drink it simply because they like the taste of this pleasant beverage. Now, catnip has been promoted by certain members of the counter culture as a psychedelic drug, said to produce a sense of well-being or euphoria when smoked like tobacco or marijuana. Even now, it is listed in practically all books devoted to drugs of abuse as a mild intoxicant. Although there is now no scientific evidence to support the sedative activity of catnip tea, many people do drink a cup of it at bedtime in the belief that it will ensure a good night's sleep.

Scull-cap is one that is also worthless, but has been praised as an excellent herb for almost any nervous system malfunction. Not only is the lack of therapeutic activity a problem associated with the use of scull-cap, but also a report in the medical literature summarized the observed heputotoxic (liver-damaging) effects of the herb in four women who had been consuming proprietary products supposedly containing it for the relief of stress. This report raises another concern, namely, the identity of scullcap. Studies in Britain showed that many wholesalers there were substituting a species of Teucrium (germander) for scullcap. Two cases of poisoning from scullcap, including one that was fatal, was reported from Riks Hospital in Oslo, Norway, in 1991. Still yet, deficiencies in activity, safety, and quality as a whole make scullcap a good herb to stay away from.

Another herb that is used to treat a host of maladies is kelp. Kelp in the form of a powder or tablets is used in folk medicine to treat constipation, bronchitis, emphysema, asthma, indigestion, ulcers, colitis, gallstones, obesity, and disorders of the genitourinary and reproductive systems, both male and female. It is also claimed to clean the bloodstream, strengthen resistance to disease, overcome rheumatism and arthritis, act as a tranquilizer, combat stress, and alleviate skin diseases, burns and insect bites. One of the advocated used of kelp is to control obesity. Claims are also made that iodine - containing kelp is useful as a blood vessel cleanser in the treatment of atherosclerosis. Many of the other medicinal uses of kelp are dependent on its content of Algin (sodium alginate). Kelp should be avoided due to its iodine and Algin content. It should be avoided because it is said to taste bad.

As I speak of another herb that is considered to have curative properties, please be aware to list it's said ability to treat a variety of ailments; would be a lengthy one. It is said to loosen phlegm, expel gas, relieve colic and for its calmative effects. Fennel has been reported to increase milk secretion, promote menstruation, and increase libido. There is no question to the safety of the fennel fruit and fennel oil. Fennel fruit itself, in quantities, is normally utilized for medicinal teas or similar preparations, is innocuous except for producing a rare allergic response. Fennel - volatile oil is a very different matter. Herbal use of fennel should be restricted.

We are always putting our faith in healing from everything other than the body. The innate wisdom of the body will heal itself as long as the cause/causes are removed. How does the weak body know to use an herb, but a well body knows not to touch it, and rid itself of it fast; as the energies of the body allows; and the body's structure is not beyond repair. No one wants to stop sinning; they just want to cover their sins. It would prove more intelligent to learn correct food combining than to have to use aloe, barberry, broom, fo-ti, horehound, pokeweed, and seana as a laxative; calamaus, carpsicum, catnip, celery seed, chamomile, dandelion, gentian, ginger, and goldenseal as a digestive or gastric aid; betony, raspberry, savor and witch hazel for gastrointestinal toxicity; angelica, capsicum, catnip, celery seed, chamomile, fennel, juniper, lovage, parsley, penny royal, peppermint, and savory for flatulence.

How does the weak body know to use an herb to make itself well? What makes the strong body, not use an herb, but proves itself dangerous in many cases. A strong person's body has high nerve energy, but the weak person's nerve energy is low. The herb is introduced to the body as a 'cure' for its dis-ease, but the body recognizes it as a poison. Toxic accumulation leads to death, so the body will attempt to rid itself of it as fast as the powers of life will allow. If the energy is high, it will reject and expel it fast. If the powers of life are low, its rejection and expulsion of waste and toxins will be slow and lead to death.

Herbs are no more than diluted drugs. Regardless of the regulatory or legal advantages that may be gained by calling them something else, whenever herbs are used to diagnose, cure, mitigate, treat, or prevent disease, they are, by definition, drugs. They do not possess any magical or mystical properties, and like other drugs, they must be administered in proper doses for appropriate periods of time to produce their benefit. These benefits result from the presence of one or more toxic principles, usually complex compounds that are present in the plant material. Every herb has a different level of toxic effect. Some are less toxic than others are. Herbs can even produce undesirable side effects.

The market for herbal medicine has exploded in the last 30 years beyond anyone's wildest expectations. Herb products intended for health benefits were once relegated to health and natural food retail outlets in the United States. Since then, herbs and herbal products have found their way into every conceivable retail outlet where non-prescription drugs and personal care products are sold, including independent pharmacies, chain pharmacies, discount department stores, supermarkets, and even checkout counter displays at convenience stores. Buyers for chain drugstores or discount department store pharmacies have filled shelf space with herb products before a new generation of pharmacists has had an opportunity to learn of the risks, benefits, proper dosage forms, co-indications, and side effects of the thousands of herb products that have flooded the market. No matter how we try herbs, dietary supplements, fairy dust, or healing potions, herbs are still drugs. A pharmacist selling herb products or advising consumers on product benefits that milk thistle fruit extracts standardized to 80% percent solitarian, may be beneficial for certain liver conditions. He or she should also know that there is not one shred of evidence to suggest that therapeutic benefit can be expected from powdered milk thistle leaf products, in whatever form they are sold.

The rebirth of the herbal cure is a destructive one. It is one that should have died with no hope of a resurrection. You have a multitude of advocates who put their trust in these herbal poisons. More students are now following academic career paths toward a pharmacognosy degree. There is a high chance that all medical schools in the United States offer at least undergraduate programs in so-called alternative or complementary medicine. Even with the herbal toxic nature, the murderous thugs from the medical mentality sees the folly in them as does the herbal society sees the folly in the medical mentality, but now see that their mentality is actually the same. Both schools of healing looks to cure or force the body by forced stimulation. None removes the cause of the ailment or applies hygienic means to restore health to the individual. Herb products are much more widely available, offered more often than not repackaged by marketing companies with no internal scientific knowledge of the substances they purvey, truth can indeed be stranger than fiction.

I have watched many individuals go in and out of numerous drugstores buying different types of herbs. We are told that we should use grape seed extract for our medical woes, but we are encouraged to spit the seeds out as we eat grapes. Our vegetables are said to be better peeled. We are an ignorant generation by believing that we can get a better health benefit from a denatured food extract over the whole food itself. The ideal diet is one of fresh fruits, vegetables, nuts, and seeds eaten in a modest amount while in an emotional balance. These things should be eaten whole and raw.

The information is supplied by the health books, health food store deals, and different quantities of promotional literature. The promotional literature on these modern herbals range from small, cheaply printed, paper-covered pamphlets dealing with single or, at most, small groups of drugs to large, elaborately produced, comprehensive studies in fine blindsiding with attractive artwork and numerous color plates. Most of them all apply some sort of strategy to lure in an obvious attempt to cultivate the interest of drug abusers, emphasize plant substances with mind-altering properties. Many of the information now are found on the Internet, which provides the opportunity for a medicine show on every home computer.

When we type in a single herb in the search on the Internet, we find that we may retrieve over a thousand different web links on it. Most, if not all, offer promotional literature for products, but the task is to be able to discern between the fact and fiction. Practically, all non-scientific literature recommends large numbers of herbs for the treatment of a variety of ailments based on hearsay, folklore, and tradition. Most literature recommends everything for anything.

It is ridiculous to believe that an herb is beneficial just because it is from nature or natural. We even tend to misuse other terms in our promotional literature such as organic and health foods. Belladonna and tobacco leaves can be grown organically, but will still kill the person or persons that consume a salad bowl full of them. Man must learn that everything that is on earth is not for him to consume. He is only exhausting the powers of life.

The placebo effect is more healthful than the herbal practice. But still yet, the placebo effect will not cause removal, only the obedience to the natural laws of life will prove most healthful. "Placebo" comes from the Latin, "I will please" and refers to a drug that provides relief for the patient through mental processes rather than through any physiological effect on the disorder. Its pretty much mind over matter. A placebo does for you what you think it will do. Studies actually show that they work about one-third of the time they are used. They have been found to be effective for the relief of severe postoperative wound pain, cough, drug-induced mood changers, angina pain, headache, seasickness, and the common cold in an average of 35% of these patients. Most of the conditions for which herbal treatment is commonly used, fell into the categories of: change of behavior, subjective sensation, response controlled by the endocrine glands or by the autonomic nervous system. An herb is going to have either a placebo effect all the way to any extremely toxic effect. When we look at homeopathy, we find that the less taken is best for health. Then, we find that the smallest dose would be no dose at all. We would be wise to learn that the body is equipped with an onboard healing mechanism that does all its own repair work as needed as fast as the powers of life permits.

All therapeutic claims to herbal remedies stem from our fathers and mothers. This behavior is instilled in us from what we learn from our teachers of life. We see them put all their trust in all these shaman voodoo practices, in hopes to restore themselves to health, but only to see them fall deeper into their sicknesses and ailments. We know that soon we will be beaten on the altars of our parents gods' - looking for a pardon to our sins to only be given an illusion that appears to bring health. Our parents "gods' - become ours as we begin our worship and devoted services to them as they lead us to our early death. We must put our faith and trust into the healing powers of the body. If something is not a food and is non-usable, the body will waste valuable energy and time neutralizing and eliminating it. This neutralizing and abnormal eliminating diverts the powers of life from house cleansing to act on the poison. The more energy is diverted, the more toxic the herb is; the more poisonous substances taken from the plant, those cure mongers will claim curing, as the body's energy is diverted from healing to neutralizing, when in fact it is hindering the healing process from house cleansing. We have gone from one miracle herb that has failed to another miracle herb that will soon be known as a failure. It would be wise for this generation to learn from the mistakes of the many generations before it.

Chapter Seven

~ Imma Care for Myself ~

It has been a blessing to come into the knowledge of true hygiene. There have been many alternative health care themes that have been a part of my life for a long time, but all fell short of true hygienic health. The health program has definitely instilled in me the solid foundation needed to know in finding the true cause of disease, the reversal of disease, and how to change my life by changing my thought process. No other healthcare path is so direct and to the point. I've never been so excited and hungry to soak up all the information I could receive from this program. It's a joy to share it with family and friends, and that's done on a constant basis.

Before I started this program of care, I had the belief that conventional medicine was proven based science. I figured these doctors studied so long they must be experts in medicine. They spoke in fancy doctor talk in there white coats asking about symptoms. After they check for symptoms, they would prescribe a pill, some kind of tonic or some conventional therapy. The symptoms, in most cases, would always get worse. Only after I learned the true cause of disease did I lose the medical mentality. Toxemia is the cause of disease. This occurs when the blood becomes toxic or poisoned. There is no such thing as only part of the body is affected by toxemia; because as it runs in the blood, the toxins travel throughout the body with the blood. The weaker organs are the ones to break down first. A lot of the time the waste is stored in out of the way places, such as: joints, arteries, fatty tissue, tumors and cysts. If the toxins are in the joints, it's usually called some type of arthritis. Wherever the toxins accumulate at is often how the disease or illness is named. There are two sources of toxemia: there's endogenous toxins, there's exogenous toxins. Endogenous toxins are toxins that are created from within the body by metabolic waste, spent debris from cellular activity, dead cells, emotional and mental distress and excess, and physical fatigue or stress. Some endogenous toxins cannot be avoided in order to maintain homeostasis. Exogenous toxins are toxins that are introduced to the body from without. Exogenous toxins come from unnatural food and drink; natural food destroyed by cooking, refining, and preserving, incorrect food combining; drugs of any kind; environmental, commercial, and industrial pollutants; impure air and water. Exogenous toxins can be controlled by the individual. The toxic overload is the result of the "Energy Robbers". Internal and external uncleanliness, unclean air, impure water, inadequate rest and sleep, SAD diet, inadequate sunshine and light, abnormal temperatures, lack of exercise, emotional unbalance, and toxic relationships are the energy robbers. There are seven stages of disease. During stage one, the nerve energy is reduced or exhausted that all normal bodily functions are greatly impaired. Stage two, occurs when the nerve energy is too low to eliminate endogenous and exogenous toxins. Stage three is irritation as the toxic build-up within the blood lymph, and tissues continue. Stage four brings on inflammation, which is leading to the death of cells. During stage five, the tissues are destroyed. Stage six is induration or hardening, and seven, being irreversible cancer. Metabolism is the building up and tearing down of the body. When metabolic processes are hindered or slowed by toxins, diseases occur as a means of healing. Bad health is the result of unhealthy living conditions supplied to the body. To change health, we first have to change the medical mentality on it.

I was instructed by a medical doctor some years back: I would have to live with diabetes and my high blood pressure. It was said that even though I could not cure these problems, I could take medication to help me lead a normal life. There was always a new drug out to try. Hygiene shows how to remove the cause and symptoms of disease (toxins) from the individual's life. When nerve energy is lowered so that metabolic and digestive elimination is hindered, toxicity will accumulate very rapidly. The health program teaches you how to enhance nerve energy with pure language. To enhance is to stop robbing. Keeping the body and hair washed, the nails clean, teeth brushed, and free from internal toxic build-up. Pure air is an essential nutrient. So when the air we breathe is fresh and pure, it brings life to the body. If the air is filled with poisonous gas from pollution, it robs nerve energy supply. Pure water is necessary for vibrant health.

To be alive one must have life, and that life will be governed by physiological laws of life. Life's Great Law states that every living cell of the organized body is endowed with an instinct of self-preservation, sustained by an inherent force in the organism called "vital force" or "life force" or "nerve energy". Then you have the Law of Order, The Law of Action, The Law of Power, Law of Distribution, Law of Conservation, Law of Limitation, Law of Special Economy, Law of Vital Accommodation, Law of Dual Effect, Law of Repose, Law of Selective Elimination, Law of Utilization, Law of Quality Selection, Law of Minimum, and Law of Development. Natural Hygiene hold that health is the normal state of all living organisms and that health is maintained through natural, self-initiating, self-healing processes.

Ideal foods are those foods that are suitable for the body and doesn't cause poisons or toxins to build up. These foods must also be eaten in a combinable way to not cause digestive problems. There are three classes of enzymes: metabolic enzymes, which run our bodies; digestive enzymes, which digest our food; and food enzymes from raw foods, which start food digesting. Digestive enzymes have only three main jobs: digesting proteins, carbohydrate, and fat. Whenever raw food enzymes are ingested, it takes more of the burden off of the organism's own enzyme resource. When enzymes are destroyed through such means as cooking, refining, and processing; it forces the organism to produce more enzymes, thus enlarging digestive organs, especially the pancreas. When an excessive amount of digestive enzyme is made, the enzyme potential may be unable to produce an adequate quality of metabolic enzymes to repair the body's organs and fight disease. The only way to get enzymes from food is to eat raw food. By using more food enzymes, less digestive enzymes will be produced. This will cause the body to focus more of its attention on metabolic enzymes.

The human digestive tract was not designed by nature to digest complex meals. If we make a habit of eating complex meals and disregarding our enzymic limitations, that abdominal stress will become chronic. Food is that material which can be incorporated into and become a part of the cells and fluids of the body. Protein foods are those that contain a high percentage of protein in their make- up. Carbohydrates are the starches and sugars. Fats are all fats and oils. Fruits are acid fruits, sub-acid fruits, sweet fruits, melons and non-starchy and tender green vegetables is ideal human diet. When these are not combined in an appropriate manner, digestion is impaired. Acids and starch combinations should be eaten at separate meals. Protein-starch combinations should also be eaten at separate meals. Protein requires an acid medium. When the protein is present the carbohydrate is being ashed or burned instead of digested. Protein- protein combinations are not advised because of their different character and composition. Other and different food factors call for different modifications of the digestive secretion and different timing of the secretions in order to digest them efficiently. Proteins and acids should be eaten separate because gastric juice is not poured out in the presence of acid in the mouth and stomach. This hinders the digestion of the proteins in the meal. A fat-protein combination should be eaten separate as well as sugar protein combinations. Sugar-starch combination is not acceptable because sugar does not undergo any digestion in either the mouth or stomach, but in the small intestine only. Carbohydrate begins digestion in the mouth and continues to predigest in the pre-digestion chamber of the stomach. Now, no ptyalin is found in saliva when sugar is present. So the carbohydrates are not digested for lack of the enzyme ptyalin, and the sugars are held up in the stomach fermenting. Melons should be eaten alone, and milk also should also be eaten alone.

When milk enters the stomach it coagulates-form curds. These curds tend to form around the particles of food in the stomach thus insulating them against the gastric juice. This prevents their digestion until after the milk curd has digested. Desserts should be deserted due to its high sugar content that is held up in the stomach and doesn't get digested. Desserts are usually empty calories. They are sometimes served cold which cause your body to have to warm them up before it can start digestion. When starches and sugars undergo fermentation they are broken down into carbon dioxide, acetic acid, alcohol and water, which are all poisons except for water. When proteins putrefy or rot, they are broken down into a variety of ptomaine and leucomains, which are also poisons. To derive sustenance from the foods eaten, they must be digested and not poison us.

The dietary nature of human frugivores is evident in nature. The appeal of a slaughtered animal in a raw state doesn't compare to a ripe banana. Just the thought of eating a grape, apple, melon, peach, plum, banana, pineapple, or orange tantalizes the mind and excites the taste buds. The psychology of us proves that we were not designed to eat flesh as a carnivore does. Our digestive organs are set up in different ways, even with different capabilities. 80/10/10 is the caloronutrient ratio in maintaining good digestion health. Fruits are the closest to that ratio somewhere around 85/7/8. The caloronutrients are carbohydrates, proteins, and fats. Eighty percent (80%) carbohydrates, ten percent (10%) proteins, and ten percent (10%) fats should make up the ratio of calories in the ideal diet. The ideal diet should be eaten in a raw state, because cooking damages the nutrients in foods. Fruits do not have to be cooked only washed and served. When proteins are cooked, it denatures the protein fusing the amino acids together with enzyme resisted bonds that preclude them from being fully broken down or digested. These undigested proteins cause joint pains and allergies in the body. When carbohydrates have to be cooked to dextrinize them, their molecules are fused into a sticky, molasses-like goo. The body can only realize perhaps 70% of the energy potential of cooked starchy foods. Heated fats interfere with cell respiration, leading to cancer and heart disease; and heating fats also reduces the functional value of their antioxidant properties. When fats are cooked they become rancid and decomposes; proteins putrefy when they decompose; carbohydrates ferment in the stomach.

The physical health of the body is not accomplished alone, because mental health plays its part as well. Stress slows or halts the digestion process. When a person is in stress, they are usually always in a fight-or-flight response mode. This causes the body to produce a lot of endogenous toxins as a by-product, and we know that toxemia is the cause of disease. Cholesterol is a stress hormone and is present in those with stress. By embracing non-toxic relationships, maintaining emotional balance, eating the ideal diet and clean thoughts can make the individual more able to deal with life stresses.

We first have to have a purpose and believe that we matter. This is easily done by challenging our thought patterns and the data that is imputed in our brains, which is called the body's computer. We all carry on a 24 hour self-talk in real time. Some of our thoughts run automatic, which are called tapes. We seldom question the thoughts we have even though our thoughts don't always tell us the truth, but if a lie goes unchallenged, it becomes the truth. Everyone must examine themselves, and we learn how to deal with love and depression by killing the ANTs, surrounding yourself with positive people, recognizing the importance of physical contact, and physical exercise.

ANTs are automatic negative thoughts that are dispiriting one after the other. With them, we need to look at the future with anxiety and pessimism. Our mind's filter looks at; ourselves, others, and the world in a negative way. These negative thoughts make us behave in a way that we bring on the negativity, but when we have positive thoughts and positive attitudes, it often helps us to radiate a sense of wellbeing. Step one in enhancing positive thought patterns is to realize that your thoughts are real. Step two is to notice how negative thoughts affect your body. Notice that every angry thought, an unkind thought, or sad thought causes your brain to release chemicals that make your body feel real bad. Step three is to notice how positive thoughts affect your body. Examine how you feel when you're relaxed breathing slowly. Step four is to notice how your body reacts to every thought you have. For step five, think of all bad thoughts as pollution. Thoughts are very powerful, and if they are negative, these negative thoughts take over. Step six is to understand that your automatic thoughts don't always tell the truth. So, in step seven, you need to talk back to them. Whenever you just think a negative thought without challenging it, your mind believes it and your body reacts to it. Step eight is to exterminate the ANTs. Whenever I notice that I am having a negative thought, I picture a trashcan in on the side of my mind. I tell the negative thought that is causing me to not be happy, but I want to be happy, so you're going to have to be placed in the trash can. Then I focus on a word that brings on a happy feeling or memory. If the thought comes back up, I picture myself slamming the lid on its head hard. There are many types of ANTs that cause problems like: always or never thinking ANT, focusing on the negative, fortune telling, thinking with your feelings, guilt beating, labeling, personalizing, and blaming.

When the blood and lymph fluids are toxic, the body's ability to eliminate waste, be it endogenous or exogenous, has become insufficient. This accumulation of toxins is what cause an unhealthy living environment within the body. The symptoms that spring from disease are merely the body eliminating it though channels that conventional medical society label as specific diseases instead of the root cause "toxemia". The body repairs itself daily; so if there is more cleaning up than messing up, then the body cannot be sick and dis-ease. There are many ways to reserve your vital energy. Fasting is one that can help by allowing the digestive organs to rest, and allow the metabolic enzyme to be dominant as to repair the body more rapidly. The health program, has opened my mind up to true health. It has shown me how to reverse disease by embracing the energy enhancers. It has taught me how to obey the laws that govern our bodies. I see no reason why I can't show others how to do the same. My life has changed drastically. I'm thinking everyone who has shared and kept this knowledge alive.